TAKE
CONTROL OF
YOUR
METABOLISM

IT'S ABOUT A HEALTHIER, BETTER YOU

AND ACHIEVE LASTING AND NATURAL

WEIGHT LOSS STARTING TODAY!

Written

By R.L.Boczko

DISCLAIMER AND LEGAL NOTICES

The information presented within this book solely and fully represents the views of the author as of the date of publication. Any slight to, or potential misrepresentation of, any peoples or companies is entirely unintentional. As a result of changing information, conditions or contexts, this author reserves the right to alter content or option with impunity.

This book does not in any way substitute for medical or psychological/psychiatric advice or recommendation. You should always consult with your doctor or other qualified professional regarding any known or suspected medical or mental condition or illness, as well as before engaging in any form of exercise or making any change to your dietary practices. You should always consult with a doctor prior to beginning any new medical regimen, including changing or introducing medications, supplements, or other therapeutic procedures. As such the author cannot assume responsibility for any outcome or effect on the reader's wellbeing or health in any way whatsoever. You should always consult with a professional if you are or think you may be experiencing any sort of health condition or disorder or disease.

This book is for informational purposes only and the author does not accept any responsibility for any sort liability, including injury, stress, strain, debility or financial loss, resulting from the use of this information.

This information is not presented by a medical or psychological practitioner and is for educational and informational purposes only. The content is not intended to be a substitute for professional medical advice, diagnosis, or treatment. Always seek the advice of your physician or other qualified health care provider with any questions you may have regarding a medical condition. Never disregard professional medical advice or delay in seeking it because of something you have read or heard.

While every attempt has been made to verify the information contained herein, the author cannot assume any responsibility for errors, inaccuracies, or omissions.

Thank You for reading this...

TABLE OF CONTENTS

*"Two roads diverged in a woods, and
I took the one less traveled by,
And that has made all the different"*
-The Road Not Taken

Introduction

Why did you pick up this book? Could it be somewhere in your heart you long for a healthier you?

If you have heard about metabolism, chances are it's in relation to weight loss. Metabolism is bigger than weight loss, though, as you will learn later on. It is about a healthier, better you.

If you require taking control and starting up your metabolism and do not have any idea how to do it, you have come to the right place. In case you have tried to speed up your metabolism before but do not see visible results, you have also come to the right place.

This book will walk you through the basics of metabolism and all that you need to do to speed up your metabolism. Enjoy the book! And don't forget to take action for getting any results you want.

As and added bonus I also put a chapter in this book to help you understand the metabolism of your children. Please enjoy, and get the most out of this book.

Let's begin to talk about how we can achieve just that!

Chapter One
YOUR METABOLISM
THE BASICS

Metabolism Defined:

Metabolism, in its most basic sense, is the body's conversion of the calories from the food you eat into energy. It is a series of chemical reactions that gives your body the energy to do what it needs to do to keep functioning and consequently, for you to keep living. Without metabolism, you would not be able to move or think. Metabolism provides energy for your body and your individual organs to work smoothly.

To better understand the importance of metabolism, think about this: if your heart stops beating, you die. Likewise, if your metabolism stops, you die - because without metabolism, you won't have the energy even to breathe, or for your heart to beat!

How Metabolism Works:

First, let us start with the act of eating. As you chew and swallow your food, it goes down to your digestive tract. Digestive enzymes then break down your food - carbohydrates to glucose, fats in to fatty acids, & protein in to amino acids. After the nutrients are effectively broken down, they are absorbed by the bloodstream and are carried over to the cells. Other enzymes and hormones then work to either convert these nutrients in to cells or building blocks for tissues or release them as an energy supply for the body's immediate use.

Metabolism Types and Components:

There are two basic metabolic processes, one is constructive, and is responsible for building and storing energy for the body. The other is destructive, though in a positive sense, as it breaks down nutrient molecules to release energy.

The constructive metabolic method is called anabolism, while the destructive method is called catabolism.

Anabolism: promotes the growth of new cells, the maintenance and repair of tissues, and the storage of energy are usually through body fat, for future use. Small nutrient molecules are converted in to larger molecules of protein, carbohydrates and fat.

Catabolism: meanwhile, is responsible for immediately providing the body energy to use. Instead of building up, it breaks down the nutrient molecules to release energy.

These two processes do not occur simultaneously but are balanced by the body.

Catabolism, in particular – though some attribute this to overall metabolism – has three components:

1. **Basal metabolism** → Some times called resting metabolism, this is the metabolism component responsible for keeping you alive by ensuring normal body functions. Even if you were bedridden the whole day, basal metabolism is still at work.

   Basal metabolism is metabolism's main component, as 60 to 70 percent of the calories from the food you eat are used for this purpose. People who want to lose weight usually aim for a higher basal metabolic rate (BMR).

2. **Physical movement** → This can range from a simple moving of your fingers to strenuous exercise. Usually 25 percent of the calories you consume go here.

3. **Thermic effect of food** → This indicates the digestion and processing of the food you take in. Normally, ten percent of the calories of the food you eat are burned through this.

Thus, taking all this into account, here is our metabolism formula:

Calories from Food = Calories Expended From Basal Metabolism (60-70%) + Calories Expended By Physical Movement (25%) + Calories Expended Digesting Food (10%)

What Affects Metabolism?

Your metabolic rate, or how fast or slow your metabolism works, is influenced by a number of factors:

1. Genetics → Yes, metabolic rate is also inherited. Sometimes this makes an entire world of difference between a person who can eat almost everything and not gain an ounce and a person who easily balloons after indulging just once.

2. **Age** →The younger you are, the faster your metabolism is. Metabolism slows down as you age. Women's metabolic rate starts falling at the age of 30; for men, decline starts later at the age of 40.

3. **Gender** → Men have a faster metabolic rate – usually 10-15 percent faster – than women because their bodies have a larger muscle mass. Muscle plays a key role in fast metabolism, as will be discussed in the chapter on exercise.

4. **Amount of lean body mass** → As already mentioned above, more muscle = faster metabolism.

5. **Diet** → Some foods will help you, some will only harm you. While timing is not everything, when you eat also greatly affects your metabolism. The difference is discussed in the chapter on eating right.

6. **Stress level** → Stress is inversely proportional to metabolism. The more stress you are subjected to, the lower your metabolism. You will better understand this when we move on to the chapter about stress.

7. **Hormones** → Specific hormones metabolize specific nutrients. How well the hormones work, then, directly affects metabolism. To a certain extent, diet and stress levels affect the hormones involved in metabolism, as you will find out later. Hormonal disorders or imbalances can affect metabolism as well.

Looking at all these factors that influence metabolism, you now probably have a general idea of what you need to do to increase your metabolism – accept the things you cannot change, and work on those that you can!

But before we get into the detailed program for firing up your metabolism, first, know what's in it for you! And find out the kind of resolve you need to achieve the level of metabolism you want.

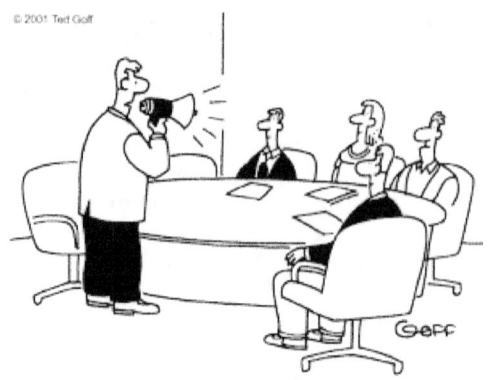

"I hope this bullhorn will make this
meeting a little less boring."

Chapter Two
WHY YOU SHOULD START UP YOUR METABOLISM

It's not all about weight loss, though discussions on metabolism seem to focus almost exclusively on this concept. In fact, even if you feel that your weight is perfectly fine, you have a lot to gain by increasing your metabolism. Following a list of the benefits you stand to gain by applying the advice in this book:

1. Lose weight - Let's start with the most obvious benefit. By increasing your metabolism, particularly your BMR, you will burn more calories just by doing the activities you usually do. Even while you lie in bed and stare at the ceiling or even while you are sleeping, your body is working to burn the calories you consume. With an increase in metabolism, you can actually shed one or two pounds a week. Best of all, the results are long-term, unlike a quick-fix diet! Now, isn't that more satisfying – and easier – than going on a fad diet?

2. **Eat more without worrying about it**

   Since you burn calories faster now, you can eat more without feeling guilty. This does not mean overindulging or snacking on junk food, though. But in general, you can be less concerned about the quantity of food you eat.

3. **Feel more energized.** People with faster metabolism report having more energy. With a faster metabolism, your body is performing efficiently to release the energy you need to get going.

4. **Look better.** The skin of people with a faster metabolism is brighter and more radiant. Their faces are pinkish, more alive with color. With a faster metabolism, you will not only feel good but also look good!

5. **Be healthier overall.** Your body functions more efficiently with a faster metabolism. Digestion, absorption of nutrients and blood circulation are improved. And you will not need as much sleep as you did before to feel refreshed the next day.

To sum it up, expect a faster metabolism to make you look and feel healthier and more wonderful.

I would like to add that as you are reading this book you will also need to follow through to get the best results. Also consult your doctor. He is trained in helping you with speeding up your metabolism.

(Use this blank page for any notes)

Chapter Three

THE RIGHT MINDSET FOR INCREASING YOUR METABOLISM

You are probably wondering what all this has to do with mindset. Why not go directly to the advice for increasing your metabolism?

The reason is that you need to be prepared for what lies ahead. Boosting your metabolism is a serious business. It is not like a quick-fix diet where you need only exert effort for a few weeks – and for some diets, even for a few days.

Boosting your metabolism is about changing your lifestyle and habits. Let me repeat it is about changing your lifestyle and your everyday habits. Though you may choose to start with small changes, you will still be changing the way of life you have become used to – and it may feel uncomfortable at first. Boosting your metabolism requires discipline and consistency in your actions. And since you are expecting long-term results, you are likewise expected to make a long-term investment.

From here on, please look at the advice I will be presenting as an entire package or program. You cannot do only some of them and still get the same results. The tips here follow the gestalt principle – the whole is greater than the sum of the parts. Trust that the components of the program all work harmoniously to deliver your desired result.

So now I want you to close your eyes and imagine yourself – really imagine! – What you will be like after this program has started to take effect on you. How will you look? How will you feel?

Then, do the same process for your expectations after three months, then six months – or even a year, if you can. Note the differences you see and feel.

It's a good idea to write down your expected outcome. This will help you get through the program, especially when you are having a difficult time sticking to the changes you previously committed to.

Congratulations! You have just begun with the end in your mind. This will greatly help you along the way to your goal of starting up your metabolism.

Chapter Four

HOW TO START UP YOUR METABOLISM

As I mentioned, please treat the advice you read here as an entire program in which you will need to apply *all* the components in order to boost your metabolism. If you skip one step you will not achieve the results that you are looking for.

First, we will talk about exercise, as this is perhaps the most crucial element in the program. Exercise done right can greatly contribute to increasing your BMR. Here, you will learn how to exercise smart, and not always hard, as some fitness programs might advise. We will be talking about the importance of building muscle mass and applying the right intensity to exercise.

The second section is about eating right – not about eating less, as some weight loss programs would advise – but eating smart. You will learn that the results you get will not only come from the food you eat, but *how* and *when* you eat as well.

The next section is about coping with stress. Some might see little importance in this section. Know, however, that stress is a real and strong impediment to boosting your metabolism. Bear this in mind as you read through this section.

As a added bonus in the last chapter, I also threw in on Knowing your Children's Metabolism & Weight. With all the talk of our country's problem of our children's obesity. I though it be useful for the whole family to get involved.

Take time to absorb each piece of advice. You can start applying the advice here little by little, but with the intention of putting it all together once your body has adjusted.

Fast Metabolism Fuel #1:
EXERCISE SMART

Notice that I mentioned *smart,* not *hard.* Though some exercises here may be high-intensity and may indeed be hard for you, you need not work as long and as hard as you may think. The goal here is to fire up your metabolism with an exercise program that takes the shortest time and the least effort possible without sacrificing results.

The two elements in this exercise program are strength and resistance training for building lean muscle mass and interval training for speeding up the metabolic process in general.

Strength and resistance training

The exercises under this training program are designed to literally build strength and resistance, as the name suggests. Tension is applied on the muscles to achieve this. The end result is increased muscle mass in your body.

Building muscle is important as more muscle in your body means more calories burned. Fitness trainer and consultant Robert Reames gives a perfect analogy by calling muscles fireplaces in the body that burn fuel – meaning calories. So the more fireplaces, the more fuel burned. For every pound of muscle added to your body, 40-50 calories more are burned per day.

Women need not worry about gaining large, unsightly muscles – your bodies are different from men. Your muscles will only add definition to your shape and in fact, make you look sexier.

While building muscles are usually associated with weight training, this is not always the case. There are in fact several exercises that do not require weights at all. If you are on a tight budget, you can in fact do exercises with no weights at all. For best results, though, do a combination of strength exercises with equipment and without equipment.

For clear differentiation, let us discuss weight lifting exercises first.

Weight lifting- is a convenient muscle-building exercise as it applies tension to your muscles through an external source, the weights. You can also easily measure your progress as the number of pounds or grams is indicated on each weight. As your body adjusts and strengthens, you can add more weights or replace your current weights with heavier ones.

To determine how many grams or pounds your weights should have, try them out first. The best weights for you are those that put tension in your muscles but do not make you feel fatigued.

The best exercises for achieving faster results for boosting metabolism are those that work several muscles in your body together. It's not a problem if you want to focus on a particular muscle, though, for example, if you want to tone or sculpt a specific body part.

There are many weight-lifting exercises you can choose from to include in your routine, but here are some basic examples:

1. **Bench press** – This is a multi-joint exercise, working the major muscles of the shoulders, chest and triceps. To do this, lie on a bench and hold the weight over your chest with your elbows bent at 90 degrees. "Press" the weight up until your arms straighten, then lower it slowly back to your starting position.

2. **Chest fly** – This works the chest, with an emphasis on outer muscles. Lie on a bench with your weights held overhead, palms facing inward. Lower the weights to your sides up to shoulder level, with your elbows slightly bent. Slowly bring the weights up, back to starting position.

3. **Bicep curl** – This is one of the most basic weight lifting exercises. This puts effort on the biceps, as the name suggests. To do this, hold the weights with your palms facing out. Bend your elbows to bring the weights to your shoulders without touching them. Slowly lower the weights down, but do not straighten the arm out totally to keep a level of tension.

4. **Concentration curl** – This also works the biceps. Kneel on one leg using the leg opposite the hand you are working with. Hold one weight with your working hand and put the other hand on your waist. Place the back of the upper arm of your working hand on the inner thigh of the other leg. You can lean into that leg to raise your elbow a little. Raise the weight to the front of your shoulder and then slowly lower the arm until almost straight.

5. **Overhead press** – This works the shoulder muscles. Stand or sit straight and hold your weights with your elbows bent and your hands in front of your eyes. Bring the weights over your head while keeping your back straight. Slowly bring the weights down to starting position.

Strength exercises without weights can be combined with weight lifting exercises for your routine.

Here are some examples:

1. **Squat** – A squat is a multi-joint exercise working the hamstrings, quadriceps, gluteals, and the lower back. In fact, this is one of the most effective strength exercises without weights. From a standing position, slowly lower your body until your knees bends at a 90-degree angle. Keep your feet flat on the floor while doing this. Return to a standing position slowly as well.

2. **Pushup** – This is also a very typical but effective strength and resistance exercise. While the basic one works well, adding complexity can work more muscles.

For example, you can do pushups between two chairs. These work the chest and the triceps. Place both feet on a stable chair and then place both hands on separate chairs. The two chairs your hands are resting on can have a gap of 60 centimeters. The chair with your feet should align with the middle of the other two chairs. Your body should be stretched naturally from the chair at your feet to the chairs in front. Slowly bring your chest down – beyond the surface of the chairs if you can!

3. **Crunch** – Yes, the basic crunch is a strength exercise, although it works mostly for the abs only. But though the crunch is well-known, not everyone knows how to do it properly. To do this correctly, lie on the floor or a mat with your knees bent and your feet flat on the floor. You may put your hands behind your head. Raise your upper body – but lead with your chest – upwards until you feel your abs contract. To keep the tension, do not raise your body up to 90 degrees. Again, to keep tension, when you bring your body down, do not let it rest on the floor. Instead, keep yourself a bit elevated from the floor.

, For variety in exercises and for working different sets of muscles, you can also try working out with different equipment like exercise balls.

In planning your routine for strength exercises, refer to the body's muscle groups below and determine which you want to work on. Remember though, that multi-joint exercises are still best to achieve faster metabolism.

1. **Biceps** – These are found at the front of your upper arm.

2. **Triceps** – These are at the back of your upper arm.

3. **Deltoids** – These are the caps of your shoulders.

4. **The Pectoralis major** – This is the large, fan-shaped muscle on the front of your upper chest.

5. **Rhomboids** – These are muscles in the middle of your upper back and located between the shoulder blades.

6. **Trapezius** – This is on your upper back, sometimes called 'traps.' The upper trapezius, in particular, runs from the back of your neck to your shoulder.

7. **Latisimus dorsi** − These are large muscles that go down the middle of your back. When exercised well, they give your back an attractive V shape, giving the illusion of a smaller waist.

8. **Lower back** − This comprises the erector spine muscles that enable back extension. This also helps in maintaining good posture.

9. **Abdominals** − Of course! This is where the belly fat usually goes, the flab you want to banish forever. The abdominals are composed of the external obliques, which trace paths down the sides and the front of the abdomen, and the rectus abdominus, a flat muscle running across the abdomen.

10. **Gluteals** – Also called "glutes," the main muscle here is the gluteus maximus, the muscle on your buttocks.

11. **Quadriceps** – These muscles go up the front of your thigh.

12. **Hamstrings** – These are on the back of your thighs.

13. **Hip abductors and adductors these** are located at your inner and outer thigh. Abductors are on the outside, moving the leg away from your body. On the other hand, adductors are on the inside, pulling the leg to the center of your body.

14. **Calf** – The calf muscles are on the back of the lower leg. The two calf muscles are the gastrocnemius and the soleus. The former gives the calf a stable, round shape while the soleus is a flat muscle below the gastrocnemius.

After choosing your exercises, you must think about the level of intensity and the duration of your exercises. The number of repetitions and sets actually depends on your level of tolerance – fatigue is a sign that you have overtaxed yourself. Let yourself feel the "burn" in your muscles or the soreness but do not push yourself more than you can go. In general, though, the American College of Sports Medicine recommends three sets or more of strength exercises with six to eight repetitions for each set for building muscle. If you are a beginner, though, it may take time before you reach this level. Not more than a 45-second rest should be taken between sets for best results in increasing metabolism.

Your exercise routine can last for only 30 minutes or less and still achieve optimum results.

At this point, I want to emphasize that strength and resistance exercises are the best *and* healthiest way to build muscles. Do not ever look for shortcuts, like performance-enhancing drugs or steroids with growth hormones. While they may help increase your muscle mass, they can have side effects such as heart attacks, liver damage, and even premature death. It is best for you to stick to the healthy and proven methods in building muscles.

The benefits of strength exercises are also numerous and not merely confined to boosting metabolism. They lower blood pressure, improve balance and flexibility, increase your stamina for other activities, and reduce your risk of injury – as these are *strength* exercises, they in fact strengthen your muscles and bones!

Interval training

Yes, these exercises are about "intervals," particularly the intervals of high-intensity exercise and rest. In this training, you do a cardiovascular exercise at the highest intensity you can manage, then shift to a moderate intensity, do high intensity again, and then moderate, and so on. Reames calls this "metabolic burst" training, as the sudden burst you do in the high-intensity exercise also results in a burst of calorie-burning. Because of the sudden "burst" you give to your body, it also suddenly releases energy. The rest period, meanwhile, is essential for the body to get rid of the waste products in the muscles you are using in the exercise. It is important to keep a moderate intensity of exercise and not go into total rest. This is to ensure that the release of energy is continuous.

Interval training can be done for almost any type of cardiovascular exercise – running, biking, swimming, and more. For running, the rest period can be brisk walking; for biking and swimming, the activity can be done at a slower but moderate pace. The high-intensity and moderate-intensity exercise can also be slightly different. For example, the high-intensity exercise may be briskly walking up the stairs while the low-intensity exercise may be brisk walking on a flat surface.

Each interval should last between one to four minutes. The rest period can be shorter or longer than your high-intensity exercise, depending on your condition. Doing your interval training routine for a total of 30 minutes already achieves optimal results. Just ensure that your moderate-intensity exercise really still *has* intensity while allowing your body to rest for the next burst of high-intensity exercise. Perform your personal best for the high-intensity exercise – being almost out of breath is a good sign.

A more accurate way of determining the highest level of intensity you can manage is by calculating your maximum heart rate. To get your maximum heart rate, simply subtract your age from 220. During exercise, a heart rate monitor will come in handy although this is optional. To monitor your heart rate manually, find your pulse in your wrist then count the number of beats within six seconds. Put the number zero at the end of that. If you counted 16 beats, your pulse rate is 160 beats per minute. Your pulse rate after high-intensity exercise should be 75-85 percent of your maximum heart rate. Your pulse rate during moderate-intensity exercise should always be greater than your resting heart rate or your normal heart rate when you are not doing any exercise. Again, to get your resting heart rate, get your pulse rate while you are not doing exercise.

For those who want to boost metabolism primarily to lose weight, here's the good news: after a few weeks of interval training, expect even your normal exercise with moderate intensity to burn more fat than usual.

A study by exercise scientist Jason Talanian supports this claim. After seven interval workouts distributed over two weeks, subjects increased their fat burning by 36 percent through normal cycling exercises only.

Also, according to Reames, after interval training comes the "metabolic afterburn" – this means that your body continues burning calories for *46 hours* after your workout.

Interval training sure beats normal cardiovascular training. Also, normal cardiovascular exercise usually takes longer as the objective is endurance. Contrast this with interval training which only requires 30 minutes or less and which delivers significant results in just a few weeks.

Putting it all together

While you will be choosing your specific exercises for the strength and resistance training and interval training, I will be recommending an exercise schedule and giving you tips for your best application of the exercises.

Below would be the best weekly schedule for your workout:

Day 1: Strength and resistance exercises

Day 2: Interval training exercises

Day 3: Strength and resistance exercises

Day 4: Interval training exercises

Day 5: Strength and resistance exercises

Day 6: Interval training exercises

Day 7: Rest

As you can see, strength exercises and interval training are done on alternate days. This is to facilitate recovery of the muscles you use. Do not ever, ever does your strength exercise workout right after your interval training workout – this will slow down the process of muscle building.

One day without exercise during the week is also crucial for your body to make a full recovery.

Again, I would like to emphasize that you should never push your body to fatigue. Doing so would trigger a stress response in your body, which may have serious effects on your metabolism. (The link between stress and metabolism will be discussed in a later section). Also, make sure that you breathe normally throughout the exercises so that your body is not stressed.

Always perform warm-up exercises before your routine and cool-down exercises after. For a warm-up, a cardio of moderate intensity and arm circling would be a good example. For a cool-down, a total body stretch will relax your muscles. Breathing exercises will also help in relaxing.

You can apply variety to your exercise routines to work different muscles and for your own enjoyment, especially if you get bored with the same exercise routines.

Metabolism Checkpoint:

Before we proceed...

Here are some more things to think about as you plan your exercise program to start up your metabolism:

1. **Age does not matter.** Yes, whether you are 20 or 60, you can trust that the exercise program we discussed will work for you. For older people, your interval training may not be as intense at first, but after some time, you just might be surprised how far your body can go. Looking at strength and resistance training in particular: here's something for older people to consider: a scientific study conducted at Tufts university shows that age is not an obstacle to building muscle. In their study, 87 to 96 year-old women who underwent an 8-week strength training program tripled their strength and increased their muscle by ten percent.

2. **Other exercise is good, but...** I recommend you apply the exercise program discussed here. While it is true that any physical activity burns calories, it only has a one-time effect. The exercises here, however, are guaranteed to have a long-term effect. Also, endurance training is good, but you will get more and faster results from interval training.

3. **More exercise does not mean faster metabolism.** Logically, more exercise means more calories burned. But as your goal here is a long-term increase in your metabolism, you should not be obsessed by how much you exercise but on the quality of your exercise. Again, this deserves repetition – do not push yourself beyond your limits as it will drive your body into a stress reaction. Stress has a serious effect on metabolism.

"Great men are they who see that
The spiritual is stronger then
Material force, that thoughts rule
The world."
-Ralph Waldo Emerson

So now you know the best exercise program to start up your metabolism. But don't stop reading just yet – exercise is only one part of your journey to a faster metabolism.

(Use this blank page for any notes)

Fast Metabolism Fuel #2:
EAT RIGHT

Food is your main fuel for energy – it gives your body the calories it processes to burn or to store energy. The right food, the right amount, and the right time in eating will give you the best results possible for your metabolism.

For all those who are trying to lose weight, you need to know that eating to boost metabolism is radically different from traditional weight loss diets. In traditional diets, calories are your enemy and you have to monitor your calorie intake, but the opposite is true for the fast metabolism diet. Calories are now your friends – the good calories, at least.

Remember when we talked about exercise? The more muscles you build, the more calories you burn. And after you've done interval training for a while, your body also burns more calories. So to keep up with the calories burning, you actually have to eat more. You will understand this better later.

Nutrients to Befriend

Carbohydrates are one of the most essential nutrients for starting up your metabolism. They are the most basic fuel for the energy you consume for physical activities. If you exercise regularly, carbohydrates are necessary. But if you are building muscle, carbohydrates are *crucial*. As you progress in your muscle building and interval training, you need to increase your carbohydrate intake. As your body burns more energy, it will need more energy from carbohydrates. If the carbohydrates you consume are not enough, your body will turn to your muscle mass and get its energy there. Yes, your hard-worked muscles will be wasted if you do not consume enough carbohydrates.

More than 50 percent of your calorie requirements should come from carbohydrates.

There are two types of carbohydrates – simple and complex. Simple carbohydrates are easier to digest and absorb compared with complex carbohydrates. If we are to consider the thermic effect of food which also contributes to faster metabolism, complex carbohydrates are the way to go. And usually, complex carbohydrates are the healthy types of food while the simple carbohydrates are usually the processed foods loaded with preservatives and artificial sweeteners.

But simple carbohydrates should not be neglected entirely. Healthy sources of simple carbohydrates are honey, milk and fresh fruit juice.

For complex carbohydrates you have a wider range of options. See the table on the next page for some examples.

COMPLEX CARBOHYDRATES

Grains and Cereal	Root Crops	Vegetables
Oatmeal	Potato	Broccoli
Whole Wheat Bread	Sweet Potato	Cauliflower
Whole Wheat Pasta	Taro/Yam	Cabbage
Brown Rice	Manioc	Eggplant
Bran	Turnips	Cucumber
Corn		Green Peppers
		Tomatoes
		Bean Sprouts
		Squash
		Asparagus
		Garlic
		Onion

Yes, carbohydrates are not all grains and root crops. We have fibrous carbohydrates as well – the vegetables. The fiber, though not absorbed by the digestive system, helps in the thermic effect. Fiber also cleanses the body and thus ensures its smooth functioning, including the enzymes and hormones for metabolism.

Protein- is another essential nutrient in the diet for faster metabolism. Protein is processed by the body into amino acids, the building block for cells – and consequently, muscles. And, like complex carbohydrates, protein also has a thermic effect as it takes a long time for the body to break it down.

On the next page are some healthy, excellent sources of protein:

1. **Chicken** – Go for the breast, as it has the highest amount of protein. Drumsticks are also good, though not so high in protein. Just remove the skin to get rid of saturated fat and cholesterol.

2. **Fish** – This is good protein without the bad, unlike red meat. Aside from having a high protein content, it is also good for the heart, particularly coldwater fish like salmon and tuna.

3. **Eggs** – Very rich in protein and affordable too. Eggs contain all the essential amino acids for growth. Contrary to what some may think, the high protein content comes mostly from the egg white and not the egg yolk.

4. **Milk** – This is a must for anyone who wants to build muscle. It is no wonder that babies and toddlers are given milk for growth. So learn from your childhood and drink milk.

5. **Whey** – Though not a natural whole food, whey is very high in protein and is also healthy. It is a staple among body builders. Whey is sold as protein powder.

Fats are also essential for fast metabolism. Now, this may raise a few eyebrows, especially among those who have tried conventional weight loss diets. This is where the fast metabolism diet, again, sets itself apart. While too much fat – especially unhealthy fat – is bad, a small amount of healthy fats helps hormones responsible for metabolism to continue performing well. Diets low in fat lead to poor hormone production, and thus, slower metabolism.

When adding fats to your diet remember to keep them in their proper place: at the top of the food pyramid. Healthy sources of fat are olive oil, avocados, sunflower seeds, and nuts.

As with fats, **calcium** helps release hormones that boost metabolism. Milk, of course, is the best source of calcium. Yogurt is also high in calcium and has other health benefits as well.

"Nutrients" to Avoid

Avoid empty calories like the plague. These come from refined, highly processed foods – usually the simple carbohydrates that are not natural whole foods. Why empty calories? They fill you up but give little or no nutrients. What's more, these foods usually contain a lot of sugar – and too much sugar seriously affects the metabolism.

Just to drive home the point, below are examples of foods with empty calories:

Candies
Gums
Chocolate bars
Pastries
Cakes
Biscuits
Soft drinks
Fast food
Flavored drinks
White bread, rice and pasta

Too much caffeine is also not good for your metabolism. It triggers a stress response. So go easy on the coffee, even diet soda pop.

Other Recommended Foods

1. **Spices** – Cayenne pepper and red hot pepper, in particular, contain capsaicin which is said to raise metabolism up to 25 percent for three hours.

2. **Green Tea** – It's not all about antioxidants. Taken regularly, green tea can increase the thermic effect of food. Research from the University of Geneva shows that green tea speeds up fat oxidation in addition to boosting metabolism. Green tea also has less caffeine than coffee, whose caffeine level may greatly affect metabolism. For those who do not like the bitter taste, green tea extract is available in capsule form.

3. **Soy** – A study conducted by the University of Illinois shows that ingesting soy protein increases metabolism. The soy protein was injected, though, and not fed to the subjects. While the study is not 100 percent conclusive, taking soy, with its healthy protein and immunity-building properties, will not hurt.

Water is life – and fuel – for metabolism

The old advice holds true for overall health as well as metabolism – drink at least eight glasses of water a day. Dehydration affects metabolism through a drop in body temperature. This drop triggers your body to store fat to help increase or maintain your body temperature.

Also, as you will be doing more exercises, you need water to keep your energy levels. If you sweat a lot, you should drink more water – even more than the eight glasses.

Water cleanses the body of toxins and thus enables body processes to proceed smoothly, including metabolism.

Timing is key element in eating

Even though you are consuming the right foods, your results will be compromised if your timing is not perfect. Follow the advice on the next page and you will get the best results.

1. **Eat several meals a day, every two and a half hours to three hours.**

To really maximize the thermic effect of food, you need to eat more than the usual three meals. Eating every three hours will allow the thermic effect to last you throughout the day, as it takes between two and a half to three hours to digest food while protein broken down to amino acids stays for three hours in the bloodstream. For the exact number of meals, the magic number for men is six while it is five for women. Men require 600-900 more calories every day than women.

Do not go over your optimal number of meals, especially through late night snacking. When you are asleep, your body has a difficult time digesting. Also, the calories from your last meal are stored as fat. Keeping the last meal light and easier to digest compared with the earlier meals is recommended.

2. **Always eat breakfast.** Your body has been in starvation mode during your sleep time. To get your metabolism up and running again, start the day right with a healthy, hearty breakfast. The later you eat your first meal for the day, the later your metabolism starts. So I recommend 15 to 30 mins. After you wake up.

3. **Do not skip meals.** Under no circumstances should you skip meals, especially the three basic meals. If you have a busy schedule and have a hard time snacking, keep "emergency" foods within your reach, like whole wheat crackers and bananas. During particularly hectic days, just a few crackers or one banana would suffice as a snack to keep your metabolism running. A fresh fruit shake or a protein shake would also be enough.

4. **Take one snack or meal after your workout.** A meal or snack with protein and carbohydrates taken within one hour after your workout for the day helps in the recovery of your muscles and the building of new ones.

5. **Do not eat less than two and a half hours before bedtime.** Though metabolism still happens while sleeping, digestion will be difficult and your calories will most likely be stored as fat in your body.

Sample meal plans

On the next page are two sample meal plans for a day. The key in each meal, particularly the main ones, is to combine protein and carbohydrates. Portions depend on your personal daily calorie requirements. Remember, though, that carbohydrates should have the biggest share in your diet – and these include hefty servings of vegetables! – followed by protein. Calcium is also essential. Fats are the least priority. You can include green tea with your meals – six cups throughout the day is best.

MEAL PLAN 1

6 AM - Meal 1

Oatmeal with banana slivers

Poached egg

9 AM - Meal 2

Protein Shake

1 PM - Meal 3

Skinless chicken breast drizzled with olive oil

Brown rice

Steamed broccoli

4 PM - Meal 4

Green beans

Potatoes

7 PM - Meal 5

Salmon fillet

Sweet potato

Cauliflower

MEAL PLAN 2

6 AM - Meal 1

Egg white pancakes (only one or two yolks can be added)

Choice of fruit/s – banana, blueberry and/or strawberries

9 AM - Meal 2

Yogurt

Choice of fruit

1 PM - Meal 3

Vegetable curry

Brown rice

4 PM - Meal 4

Fruit salad with greens and grilled chicken

(Note: dressing should ideally be vinaigrette, with olive oil)

7 PM - Meal 5

Chili (made of turkey, kidney beans and salsa)

Steamed vegetables

Milk can be taken as a last "meal."

These meal plans are here just to give you an idea. Create your own, but remember the principles. You can also change the times here, but remember not to eat too late at night.

(Use this blank page for any notes)

Metabolism Checkpoint:

Before we proceed…

Below are just some caveats and some things to watch out for in eating and nutrition for faster metabolism:

1. **Some foods can only take you so far.** Spicy foods and green tea do have some effect in boosting metabolism, but only as an addition to a diet already rich in protein and carbohydrates. Relying on these alone for your diet for faster metabolism is not enough.

2. **Some foods won't take you there at all.** Grapefruit especially is popular among dieters as its high acidity is perceived to burn fats. However, there is no scientific proof for this.

3. **No supplement will boost your metabolism.** To those who are taking supplements to boost your metabolism, you may just be wasting your money. Again, there is no scientifically proven link between supplements and faster metabolism.

4. **Diet pills are a no-no.** For those who want to lose weight, some diet pills may burn some fat and control your appetite. However, they do NOT boost metabolism. Also, the downside of diet pills is that once you get used to a certain dose, you need to take more to get the same effect as before. A few of those diet pills out there may indeed boost metabolism, but can have serious side effects. Read the box or container carefully. Better yet, consult your doctor. Looking at the adverse effects diet pills can have, wouldn't you prefer to boost your metabolism the natural way? You will look and feel better.

We are now on the last leg of the program to start up your metabolism. Keep reading!

Fast Metabolism Fuel #3:
DE-STRESS

You might be wondering what the purpose of this section is – isn't stress supposed to be a daily, ordinary part of life? But that is just the point. We now live in a fast-paced culture driven by urgency and deadlines. The more things you get done in less time, the better. Work, family and recreation have become a balancing act. Tension, worry, anxiety and fear are all too common. Emotional problems like failure in marriages, deaths of loved ones, or simply troubled relationships are accompanied with pressures from work.

Stress, especially prolonged exposure to stress, can seriously affect your metabolism, as well as your overall health and well-being.

The stress and metabolism link

There is a hormone in our body called cortisol, which aids in certain body functions. It aids regulation of blood pressure, release of insulin for blood sugar stability, increase of immunity, and proper metabolism of glucose. Small increases of cortisol can be beneficial, resulting in a quick, healthy jolt of energy and immunity, heightened memory, and a higher pain threshold. However, when too much cortisol is released or if it is released too often, it results in the following:

Blood sugar imbalances
Higher blood pressure
Decreased immunity
Lower cognitive performance
Decrease in bone density
Decrease in muscle tissue

Cortisol particularly stimulates amino acid release from your muscles to be converted to glucose that will serve as an energy source for your body to cope with stress. Yes, your hard-earned muscles are at the mercy of cortisol if you don't control its levels in your body.

The release of cortisol is mainly triggered by stress, whether physical or emotional in nature. Remember what we talked about for your exercise routine? Do not overtax yourself as it triggers the body's stress response.

Stress is also harmful to the body as it leads to the production of more acid than the body needs. Our bodies usually have an 80 percent alkaline and 20 percent acid balance. More acid in the body will upset that balance. Too much acid decreases your immunity and makes you more vulnerable to illness. Too much acid also affects body functions, including metabolism.

You can effectively cope with stress and keep your cortisol levels healthy and stable, though. When your body goes into the stress response, it is important that you help it go into the relaxation response.

Ways to de-stress

There are many ways to de-stress, as there are many causes of stress. Pick the ones to your liking.

For "re-charging:"

1. **Aromatherapy** – This is particularly effective to let your stress during the day dissipate. Lavender and mint essential oils have excellent relaxing properties. A few drops mixed with water on your oil burner will suffice. You can also combine aromatherapy with meditation. As the aroma envelops you, feel it slowly sucking in your tiredness and worries. As the aroma leaves later on, imagine that your tiredness and worries are also going away with it. You can also briefly relax with aromatherapy during work. Put a few drops on a piece of tissue paper and inhale. Close your eyes while doing this.

2. **Massage** – This is also aptly called touch therapy. A massage is also beneficial as it loosens the muscles and joints that may have tensed up due to continuous stress. Back muscles are particularly susceptible to this. You can also combine massage with aromatherapy – you can ask the masseur or masseuse to use essential oils for your massage. Peppermint is particularly excellent. Aside from its aroma, it has a cooling effect on the body when used as massage oil.

3. **Music therapy** – Put some gentle, relaxing music on your player, sit or lie in a comfortable position, close your eyes, and let the music wash over you. Imagine it washing away your worries, fears, and anxieties. A good alternative to soothing music is the sounds of nature, like ocean waves. Recordings of nature sounds are available in music stores. If you find you enjoy relaxing on the beach, then bring the beach home with you through a recording of ocean waves.

4. **Imagery** – Imagine that you are a kite slowly rising and floating through the air. You float in the bright blue sky in perfect balance and harmony with the wind. After some time, feel yourself slowly gliding downwards and then softly touching the ground. The above imagery is particularly helpful not only for relaxing but for simulating a good response to stress – notice that the motion of the kite is in harmony with the wind, when the same wind can also make the kite spin out of control.

Another imagery technique is to imagine a beautiful scene from nature like a mountaintop, a secluded island, or a tropical rainforest. Imagine yourself, from a first-person perspective, walking through the place and taking in all the beauty.

You can vary the place you visit every time you use this technique, or you can pick one and make it your sanctuary – the place you flee to during moments of stress.

For the long-term:

1. **Think positive!** – Thoughts greatly influence your health and well-being. Your thoughts can actually manifest into reality, as maintained by philosophers, contemporary speakers and even scientists. So bad thoughts can manifest negatively, while positive thoughts manifest positively. So if you are going to think, you might as well think of pleasant things. If you have anxieties over something, like an upcoming presentation for work, imagine yourself – from the first-person perspective – giving an excellent, flawless presentation. Imagine the reactions of your audience. Feel the feelings as if you were there already. Images are more powerful than words, so apply the same principle to your thoughts.

2. **Let go of negative feelings.** Wallowing in negative feelings equals more acid in the body. No wonder tension and fear lead to heartburn or indigestion while chronic worry and or resentment makes you more susceptible to high blood pressure.

   However, do not suppress your feelings, even though some may appear irrational to you. Doing so also leads to higher acid levels in your body. Feel the feeling, express it through healthy catharsis in a safe environment if you feel the need to (e.g. screaming into a pillow) – and let it go. Yes, the key here is to let go. Do not dwell on negative feelings.

3. **Meditate daily** – Make meditation a habit. In the long term, meditation brings you peace of mind and makes you more able to cope with stress. It need not be a complex meditation – stillness and emptiness of mind is the key. Sit in a comfortable position and breathe slowly, deeply. Focus on each part of your body and feel it release its tension.

After you feel sufficiently relaxed, you can silently repeat a simple word with no particular emotional attachment for you – for example, you can say "tree." Or, you can actually say a letter, like *a*. Repeat this word or letter in your mind for about one minute. Then sit still and let thoughts come to your mind. Observe your thoughts as if you were apart from them, as though they were another person's thoughts. This is so that you do not dwell on any thought. Just objectively, naturally, allow any thought to enter your mind then leave. If you reach a state of emptiness, where you feel you are thinking about *nothing*, congratulations! It may take some time for you to reach this point, though.

4. **Take up yoga.** Not only is this an excellent stress-buster, it also directly starts up your metabolism. The endocrine system and the thyroid help regulate metabolism. Yoga has many positions which give a healthy twist and compression to your

endocrine organs, thereby strengthening them for metabolism.

For relaxation from stress, though, a good yoga position is the corpse pose. As its name instructs, you should lie like a corpse. Release all tension from your body. The corpse pose is actually a good ending to your yoga routine.

5. **Plan ahead** – If the cause of your stress is recurring, plan ahead. After you have identified the cause of your stress, ask yourself if there is any way you can avoid it. For example, one cause of your stress may be the morning rush-hour traffic. To be relaxed while you are on your way to work, you have to leave early. Then you remember you watch television every night, sometimes late into the night. To avoid stress in the morning, you conclude you can decrease your television time and go to sleep earlier the night before.

By the way, if your body is subjected to stress such as long working hours, you should modify your diet while still keeping the principles of the fast metabolism diet. You especially need Vitamin C, as this helps the body cope during stress. Load up on citrus fruits and strawberries. For vegetables, sweet red pepper is an excellent source of Vitamin C. Other than that, your diet remains the same – load up on complex carbohydrates, particularly fibrous ones and take in protein.

Why sleep is important

Sleep is the time your body fully recovers from your workouts. This is also the time that your muscles grow – yes, they do not grow during your workout but while you are in bed. With little sleep, your muscles grow very little even if you put in much effort in your workouts.

Lack of sleep will also prevent your body from being in top form and will thus also affect your energy for workouts. You might find yourself getting tired easily even after a few sets or reps.

Also, scientific studies show that lack of sleep affects carbohydrate metabolism. Glucose is not metabolized as much, resulting in increased hunger and decreased overall metabolism.

It is important for you to get at least eight hours of sleep every night for the body to fully re-charge for the next day. Although people's circadian rhythms may differ, the normal circadian rhythm is 10 pm to 6 am. This is the best period for muscles to grow. So sleep early to increase your metabolism!

Metabolism Checkpoint:
Before we proceed...

For some, de-stressing may be the most difficult part of the program to boost metabolism. What if stress has become a lot of elements, of your everyday life that making serious changes in your lifestyle is difficult? You can take things slowly. The least you require to do, though, is to find some calm time to yourself every day. It can be as small as ten minutes. Use those ten minutes to relax and meditate.

Meditation goes a long way. Even ten minutes every day helps you cope better with stress. Studies show that individuals who meditate regularly are less stressed and are more able to meet life's demands. If there's occasions you cannot avoid staying up late, catch up on sleep on the weekend. Do not let your sleep "debt" accumulate. Sleep "debt" leads to poor cognitive function and poor health overall. Your body processes do not function as well as they ought to and that includes metabolism. Take time to de-stress. It not only boosts your metabolism but also improves your health in general.

So now you know the entire program. But we are not through just yet!

(Use this blank page for any notes)

Chapter Five

START UP YOUR METABOLSIM NOW!

You have learned all you need to do - now is the best time to start.

In sum, you have learned that metabolism is the process of converting calories in to energy for storage or immediate use. You now know that metabolism is an essential body function, working every second of your life, even while you are sleeping. And you now know the general metabolism formula, basal metabolism + physical activity + the effect of food, as well as what factors influence the rate of your metabolism.

Now you already have the knowledge on how to boost your metabolism:

Exercise smart:

- Build muscle through a combination of strength and resistance exercises with weights and without weights. Use exercises that work the most number of muscle groups possible. (2-3 sets, with 6-8 reps each)

- Increase calorie-burning through interval training with cardiovascular exercise. Alternate high-intensity exercise with moderate-intensity exercise. (30 minutes, with one to four minutes per interval)

- Do the two exercises on alternate days throughout the week. Allot one day for total rest with no exercise.

Eat right:

- If less is good for traditional weight loss diets, more is good for the fast metabolism diet.

- Stock up on carbohydrates and protein, as these are the driving forces of metabolism.

- Include calcium and healthy fats in your diet.

- Timing is important.
    - Always eat breakfast to kick off your metabolism for the day.
    - Eat five to six meals in a day, every two and a half to three hours. Never skip meals.
    - Drink at least eight glasses of water a day.
    - Take one snack or meal within one hour after your workout for the day.

De-stress

- Re-charge through "sensation therapy" (aromatherapy, massage and music) and imagery.

- For long-term improvement, meditate daily, take up yoga, and think positively. Do not dwell on negative feelings. Plan ahead to avoid stressful situations

Chapter Six

Over view of your Health

Almost 108 million Americans were overweight or obese in 1999. Until now, obesity continues to be a serious problem and is predicted to reach epidemic levels by the year 2020. Almost 108 million Americans were overweight or obese in 1999. Until now, obesity continues to be a serious problem and is predicted to reach epidemic levels by the year 2020. Here are some diseases that you are putting yourself in risk of if you are carrying a lot of extra pounds:

1. Heart disease

2. Stroke

3. Diabetes

4. Cancer

5. Arthritis

6. Hypertension

Losing weight helps to prevent and control these diseases.

The quick weight loss methods which have spread like fire these days do not provide lasting results. More often than not, dieting methods which involve dietary drinks, foods and supplement or pills do not work. If they do, the results are just temporary.

It is better to rely on a healthy weight loss option which will provide lifetime results. You have to set realistic goals and not expect to lose a lot of pounds in a short span of time.

Another Form of Exercise:

Leave your car if you are only going a few blocks from home; take the stairs instead of the elevator, jog, cycle or skate. Use these and other activities like home chores for adding muscle building. Make sure that you do this regularly and you will not even notice a different.

Eat healthy, drink lots of water, have enough sleep and exercise. This will give you a higher chance of a positive results and improving your health, which would result to a new, healthier you.

Chapter Seven
Knowing your Child's Metabolism

"What's the right weight for my kid?" is of the most common questions parents wonder about. It looks as if it is simple, but it is not always simple to answer. People have different body types, so no single number is the right weight for everyone.

Among kids the same height and age, some are more muscular or more developed than others. That is because not all kids have the same body type or create their bodies simultaneously at the exacted time.

Puberty & Growth Development

Not everyone grows & develops on the same schedule. In the coursework of puberty, the body begins making hormones that spark physical changes like breast development in girls & testicular enlargement in boys and spurts in height and also weight gain in both girls & boys. One time these changes start, they continue for several years. The average person can expect to grow as much as ten inches (25 centimeters) in the course of puberty before reaching full adult height.

Most children gain weight more quickly in the coursework of this time as the amounts of muscle, overweight, and bone in their bodies change. All that new weight gain can be perfectly fine - as long as body overweight, muscle, and bone are in the right proportion.

Because some children start developing as early as age 8 and some not until age 14, it can be normal for children who are the same gender, height, & age to have different weights

It can feel unusual for children to fine-tune to suddenly feeling heavier or taller. So it is perfectly normal for a infant to feel self-conscious about weight in the coursework of adolescence - lots of children do.

Figuring out your Kids BMI

The BMI formula makes use of height and weight measurements to calculate a BMI number. It's called the body mass index, or BMI. BMI is a formula that doctors use to estimate how much body fat a person has based on his or her weight and height. Though the formula is the same for adults and kids, figuring out what the BMI number means is a bit more complicated for kids.

For kids, BMI is plotted on a growth chart that makes use of percentile lines to tell whether a kid is underweight, healthy weight, fat, or fat. Different BMI charts are used for girls and boys under the age of twenty because the amount of body fat differs between girls and boys and body fat changes as your children grow.

Each BMI chart is divided in to percentiles. A child whose BMI is equal to or greater than the 5th percentile & less than the 85th percentile is thought about a healthy weight for his or her age. A child at or above the 85th percentile but less than the 95th percentile for age is thought about fat. A child at or above the 95th percentile is thought about fat. A child below the 5th percentile is thought about underweight.

Before you measure your child's BMI, you'll need an accurate height and weight measurement. Bathroom scales and tape measures aren't always precise. So the best way to get accurate measurements is by having kids weighed and measured at a doctor's office or at school.

How Does BMI Help Us

You can calculate BMI by yourself, but think about asking your doctor to help you figure out what it means. Doctors do over use BMI to evaluate a kid's current weight. They also take in to account where a kid is in the work of puberty & use BMI results from past years to track whether that kid may be in danger for becoming fat. Spotting this risk early on can be helpful because changes can be made before developing a weight issue.

Children are developing weight-related health issues historically in the past seen only in adults. Type 2 diabetes, high cholesterol, and hypertension are now often seen in overweight and obese children and teenagers. They are also more likely to be overweight as adults. And adults who are fat or overweight may create other serious medical conditions, such as heart illness.

Although BMI can be a lovely indicator of body fat, it does not always tell the full story. Someone with a large frame or plenty of muscle in lieu of excess fat (like a bodybuilder or athlete) can have a high BMI. Likewise, a tiny person with a small frame may have a traditional BMI but could still have much more body fat. These are other good reasons to speak about your BMI together with your doctor.

When Children are Overweight or Underweight

If you think your kid has gained much weight or is overly thin, a doctor ought to help you decide whether your kid has a weight issue. Your doctor has measured your child's height and weight over time and knows whether growth is proceeding right on time normally.

If concerned about your kid's height, weight, or BMI, the doctor may ask questions about your kid's health, level of physical activity, and eating habits, as well as your relative's medical history. The doctor can put all this information together to select whether there is a weight or growth issue.

If your doctor thinks your kid's weight is not in the healthy range, you will probably get specific dietary & exercise recommendations. It is vital to follow a doctor's or dietitian's plan that is designed for your kid. For kids & teenagers, significantly restricting calories or following fad diets or starvation designs can deprive them of the nutrients their growing bodies require & may well slow down growth & sexual development.

What if your kid is worried about being skinny? Most children who weigh less than others their age are fine. They may go through puberty on a different schedule than a number of their peers, & their bodies may grow and change at a different rate. Most underweight teenagers catch up in weight as they finish puberty in the work of their later teen years, & there is seldom a necessity to try to gain weight.

In a few cases, kids & teenagers can be underweight because of a health issue that needs treatment. If your child feels worn out or ill a lot, or has signs like a cough, stomachache, diarrhea, or other issues that have lasted for over a week or more, talk together with your doctor. Some kids and teenagers are underweight because of eating disorders, like anorexia or bulimia, which need immediate attention.

How Genes play an important role

Heredity plays a role in a person's body shape and weight. People from different races, ethnic groups, and nationalities tend to have different body fat distribution (meaning they accumulate fat in different parts of their bodies) or body composition (amounts of bone and muscle versus fat). But genes are not fate - kids can reach and keep a healthy weight by eating right and being active. We as parents need to assist them.

Genes are not the only things that relatives and family members may share. It is also true that unhealthy eating habits can be passed down. The eating & exercise habits of people in the same household probably have an even greater effect than genes on someone's risk of becoming overweight.

If your relatives or family eats lots of high-calorie foods or snacks or doesn't get much exercise, your children may tend to do the same. The nice news is these habits can be changed for the better. Even small changes, like cutting back on sugary drinks & going for a walk after dinner, can add up to make a actual difference. You can make it a Family type thing.

So remember, it's not a specific number on the scale that's important. It's making sure that kids stay healthy — inside and out. This also will help you staying on track with you winning the war on controlling your metabolism.

Body Mass Index Chart

BMI	19	20	21	22	23	24	25	26	27	28	29	30	35	40
4'10"	91	96	100	105	110	115	119	124	129	134	138	143	167	191
4'11"	94	99	104	109	114	119	124	128	133	138	143	148	173	198
5'0"	97	102	107	112	118	123	128	133	138	143	148	153	179	204
5'1"	100	106	111	116	122	127	132	137	143	148	153	158	185	211
5'2"	104	109	115	120	126	131	136	142	147	153	158	164	191	218
5'3"	107	113	118	124	130	135	141	146	152	158	163	169	197	225
5'4"	110	116	122	128	134	140	145	151	157	163	169	174	204	232
5'5"	114	120	126	132	138	144	150	156	162	168	174	180	210	240
5'6"	118	124	130	136	142	148	155	161	167	173	179	186	216	247
5'7"	121	127	134	140	146	153	159	166	172	178	185	191	223	255
5'8"	125	131	138	144	151	158	164	171	177	184	190	197	230	262
5'9"	128	135	142	149	155	162	169	176	182	189	196	203	236	270
5'10"	132	139	146	153	160	167	174	181	188	195	202	207	243	278
5'11"	136	143	150	157	165	172	179	186	193	200	208	215	250	286
6'0"	140	147	154	162	169	177	184	191	199	206	213	221	258	294
6'1"	144	151	159	166	174	182	189	197	204	212	219	227	265	302
6'2"	148	155	163	171	179	186	194	202	210	218	225	233	272	311
6'3"	152	160	168	176	184	192	200	208	216	224	232	240	279	319
6'4"	156	164	172	180	189	197	205	213	221	230	238	246	287	328

Conclusion

I hope that you found the book rewarding. Now you need to put it into your life, need to practice it on a daily bases to get any results. Many people just read a book and after just puts it on the shelve.

So there you have it. What you now need to do is "excuse-proof" your quick metabolism program to make sure you get the best results. In times when you feel small motivation, return to the scene I asked you to visualize yourself, after going through the program. Though people's bodies differ, you will most likely notice the end results in three or four weeks or even six weeks. Just keep after that healthier you...

Good luck! Cheers to a healthier, better you!

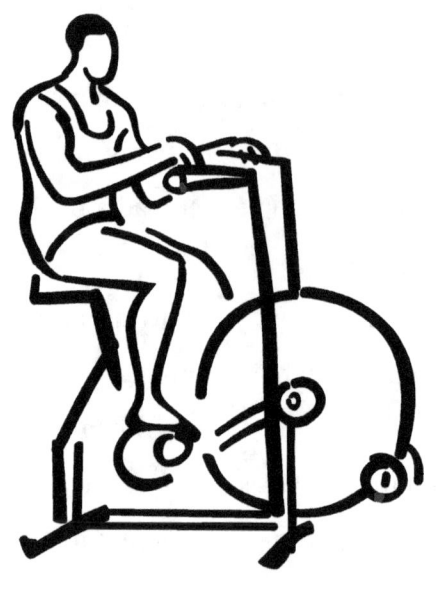

Keep working out
It will pay off in the end!

(Use this blank page for any notes)

(Use this blank page for any notes)

www.ingramcontent.com/pod-product-compliance
Lightning Source LLC
Chambersburg PA
CBHW060152290526
45789CB00003B/1012